ASCULAPIUS,
Your
Owner's Manual

ASCULAPIUS,
Your
Owner's Manual

A great little book:
The Key to healthy living

J H MILLAR

iUniverse, Inc.
New York Lincoln Shanghai

ASCULAPIUS, Your Owner's Manual
A great little book:
The Key to healthy living

iUniverse books may be ordered through booksellers or by contacting:

iUniverse
2021 Pine Lake Road, Suite 100
Lincoln, NE 68512
www.iuniverse.com
1-800-Authors (1-800-288-4677)

Designed and illustrated by Géraldine Cabannes.
Edited by Joanna Millar and Géraldine Cabannes.

ISBN-13: 978-0-595-39138-7 (pbk)
ISBN-13: 978-0-595-83524-9 (ebk)
ISBN-10: 0-595-39138-9 (pbk)
ISBN-10: 0-595-83524-4 (ebk)

Printed in the United States of America

YOUR
OWNER'S
MANUAL

§§§§§§§§§§§

BLOOD IS THE OXYGEN CARRIER.

Oxygen from your lungs is pumped by your heart to enable you to THINK, SEE and HEAR, and to digest your food and drink and to activate all your body functions. A minimum of 80% of oxygen in your blood is essential at all times!

Become aware of **your** body
with this common sense health manual.
It reveals how to protect one's IMMUNE SYSTEM to ensure a long and healthy

life.

ASCULAPIUS
STATES YOU ARE RESPONSIBLE
FOR SLOWING DOWN YOUR AGEING PROCESS.

As mentioned on page 9, the inspiration for Your Owner's Manual came from reading **the most amazing treatises on *Life Extension* by two American scientists,** Durk Pearson and Sandy Shaw.

We strongly recommend their book and the *Life Extension Companion.*

The *HEALTH* of our *PLANET*
is of vital importance to all and we have included some notes
from the WWF
and CLIMATE CHANGE towards the end of this book.

IT'S LATER THAN YOU THINK!
(a beautiful anonymous poem about life and time, page 62)

THIS GREAT LITTLE BOOK BELONGS TO:

_____

PUBLISHER'S NOTE

DAYLIGHT ENERGY FOUNDATION is a non-profit organization to save the ecology of the world.

DAYLIGHT ENERGY FOUNDATION
C/o J.H. MILLAR
Le Montaigne,
2 Avenue de la Madonne,
98000 Monaco

REFERENCES AND DISCLAIMER

The views expressed in this book have been gathered over a period of many years from doctors, specialists and experts from many countries.

These ideas and suggestions should not be substituted for professional advice from your doctor or health specialist.

Asculapius, son of Apollo and pupil of centaur Chiron, was known as a courageous and heroic healing physician.

Many modern physicians have adopted the caduceus as the "ancient" symbol of their profession, with its two intertwined snakes grasping a staff. In the ancient world, however, the caduceus was a symbol of Hermes, the Roman Mercury, who was primarily a messenger god linked with commerce. Asculapius' symbol was a single snake entwined around his staff—the 'Asculapian staff'.

The snake symbolized rejuvenation and healing to many ancient Mediterranean cultures.

CONTENTS

"Thirst and hunger for knowledge is the key to life."

Asculapius

ACKNOWLEDGEMENTS xv

INTRODUCTION xvii
    THE BODY: A MARVELLOUS MACHINE ....*xvii*

PART ONE: ANTI-OXIDANTS and NUTRITION TO COUNTER THE AGE-
ING PROCESS 1
    AGEING 2
    ADDITIONAL SUPPLEMENTS TO STAY YOUNG AND HEALTHY ..2
    FUEL FOR YOUR BODY: Liquids and Food 4
    DIGESTIVE SYSTEM 5
    HEALTHY EATING & WEIGHT PROBLEMS 5
    CRAMP 6
    GASTRO-ENTERITIS 6
    KIDNEY STONES 6
    INFLUENZA AND THE COMMON COLD 6
    PROSTATE 7
    YOUR IMMUNE SYSTEM 7
    OXIDATION and AGEING 12
    LUNGS 12
    OXYGEN 12
    SLEEP 13
    STRESS 13
    CHECK YOUR BLOOD PRESSURE 13
    METAL POISONING AND BLOCKED ARTERIES 14
    OSTEOPOROSIS (Brittle Bones) 17
    DHEA (Dehydroepiandrosterone) 19
    ARTHRITIS 20
    SEXUALITY 20
    TEETH 21
    SKIN CARE 22

EARS AND HEARING *23*

SINUS PROBLEMS *23*

PART TWO: MASSAGES AND PHYSICAL EXERCISES TO IMPROVE YOUR
HEALTH 24

EYES *24*

EYE MASSAGE AND EXERCISES *25*

NECK *29*

SPINE *29*

ARMS AND SHOULDERS *32*

NECK EXERCISES *32*

PELVIC FLOOR MUSCLES *33*

EXERCISES IN THE SWIMMING POOL *33*

BODY NETWORK—MERIDIANS *37*

MERIDIAN DIAGRAMS *38*

CONCLUSION 41

"IT IS LATER THAN YOU THINK", a poem *42*

USEFUL INFORMATION AND ADDRESSES *43*

SAVE FUTURE WATER *47*

ABOUT THE AUTHOR 51

ABOUT THE "ORIGINATOR" 53

ACKNOWLEDGEMENTS

The author wishes to acknowledge the forward thinking found in American journals: *Life Enhancement* and *Second Opinion.*

Books such as *Life Extension* and *Life Extension Companion* published in 1982 by two young American scientists, Durk Pearson and Sandy Shaw, have inspired ideas for *Your Owner's Manual.*

Dr. Hanss, a pneumonologist, and other specialists have contributed to useful knowledge.

The author gratefully acknowledges constructive help from Géraldine Cabannes.

Very many thanks to all their friends for all their advice.

To Johnny, his son, for sending articles on the research work of many scientists from America.

Finally to his wife Joanna, for her unflinching support during all this time.

INTRODUCTION

THE BODY: A MARVELLOUS MACHINE

YOUR BODY is the most ingeniously designed and engineered construction ever produced—an unique and marvellous, living, THINKING MECHANISM—.

For a machine to work well it needs regular on-going maintenance—in addition to FUEL (food and water).

You are responsible for planning and carrying out the CARE and MAINTENANCE of your own body, and if you do not pay attention every organ or part of your body will slowly become corroded and loaded with toxic poisons.

Your body can, and will, wear out—UNLESS **YOU** decide to slow down the damage and start repairs.

All the body systems must be kept in CHEMICAL BALANCE, that is, NEUTRAL. If you eat a large meal when you are tired after a heavy day's work, your stomach and digestive system will be unable to cope satisfactorily with the food and drink you are sending down. By the next morning your body will probably be out of balance chemically. It's your job to return the balance to chemical neutral.

So start repairing yourself now and start eating highly healthful foods and do all the exercises in this manual daily.

Remember that repairing your body does not just benefit the latter years of life. Techniques that increase life span **improve the quality of life NOW.**

For example, you can look more youthful, reduce aches and pains, increase muscular strength, improve resistance to diseases and stress, and even increase sexual and mental performance, including memory and learning capabilities.

DON'T STOP having **dreams** about **reaching your goals and continue to meet challenges**—this will stimulate the mind.

It is therefore in **your best interest to look after your body** as carefully as possible. The following chapters and advice should help you to do so.

> **IT'S NEVER TOO LATE TO DO SOMETHING**
> **ABOUT YOUR OWN AGEING PROCESSES!**

PART ONE: ANTI-OXIDANTS and NUTRITION TO COUNTER THE AGE-ING PROCESS

> As you get older it is important for your hearing, your eyes and your brain to maintain reasonable vitamin levels.

If you work in a town, you cannot help breathing polluted air. So, whenever you are not working, try breathing in as much clean, pure air as possible (i.e. countryside, mountains, ocean) away from cities and industrialized areas.

Some recommended healthy heart activities (walking, bicycling, swimming, hiking, jogging, skipping rope and roller skating) open your lungs and improve your heart because it challenges the circulatory system—increases the blood flow to the muscles and as the heart beats faster, the blood circulates more quickly, delivering extra oxygen to the muscles.

> **ASCULAPIUS suggests that**
> **a walk every day and deep breathing**
> **at night before bed is beneficial.**

AGEING

As one gets older, the same food does not benefit one in the same way that it did 10 or even 5 years earlier. Therefore it is imperative to take supplements to make up these losses—vitamins, minerals, essential fatty acids and other nutrients.

NUTRITIVE ENERGY is an essential factor in bodily nourishment. Energy is created when food is converted and absorbed into the blood stream. It has been proved that the ABSORPTION percentage of supplements by the body may vary between 10% and 50%, depending on whether you take it in liquid, powder or capsule form.

DID YOU KNOW THAT YOUR SKELETON RENEWS ITSELF EVERY 10 YEARS? Therefore, it is essential that you follow the correct diet and supplements for you.

ADDITIONAL SUPPLEMENTS TO STAY YOUNG AND HEALTHY

IMPORTANT WHEN TAKING SUPPLEMENTS:

If in doubt when taking nutrient supplements always check with a blood test which should reveal what you need and also indicate if you are taking too much of some vitamins or minerals. Never use supplements as a substitute for a healthy, balanced diet.

Remember the intake of vitamins for anti-ageing purposes is much higher than the normal recommended doses according to anti-ageing researchers—for example, the recommended dietary allowances (RDA) for vitamin C is only 75 mg for women, but most anti-ageing experts are recommending 500 mg or more. For men 1 gram dissolved in 1/3 glass of water FIRST THING every morning is considered suitable.

If 2,500 milligrams per day or more are taken, it may cause diarrhoea. It is very important to check with your doctor the recommended dietary allowances (RDA) for certain vitamins and minerals and their upper limits because **too much can cause disease.**

VITAMIN A-BETA CAROTENE: For eyes and anti-cancer protection. Found in apricots, cantaloupe melons, sweet potatoes, broccolis, and leafy green vegetables and, of course, carrots.

B VITAMINS: In the B group, Folic acid is important to combat coronary troubles and may prevent birth defects. Many people over 50 lose the ability to absorb B12 from natural food sources e.g. cooked green vegetables, cereals and wheat germ.

A combination of B6 and B12 helps digest animal protein for better maintenance of your body (nervous system, hair, skin, nails and cholesterol control), take a **B-COMPLEX supplement everyday**. A lack of Vitamin B leads to boils, whitlows, sties, rashes and other blood disorders.

VITAMIN C: The best protection against colds and influenza. TAKE ONE GRAM EFFERVESCENT IN 1/3 GLASS OF WATER FIRST THING EVERY MORNING. Also found in citrus fruits and raw leafy green vegetables (vitamins can be lost in cooking, see notes above).

VITAMIN D: One daily tablespoon of Cod Liver Oil,
LAST THING AT NIGHT is good for your skin and helps lubricate your joints. Sunshine is a significant source of Vitamin D because UV rays from sunlight trigger Vitamin D synthesis in the skin.

VITAMIN E: Helps block harmful cholesterol that can damage arteries. Sharpens the intellect. Best absorbed when coupled with Selenium. Found in oil-rich seeds such as apricot kernel or avocado. High levels risk uncontrolled bleeding.

BILBERRY: The extract is excellent for eyesight and memory.

CALCIUM/MAGNESIUM: Together they help retain bone density, reduce stress, avoid osteoporosis and provide the mechanism for muscle contraction and relaxation.

Be aware that calcium has a constipating effect, whereas magnesium acts as a laxative. Calcium and magnesium should both be taken with food. Remember that calcium can block iron absorption in the body and contribute to anaemia. Take 500 mg of Magnesium and 500mg of Calcium a day.

ZINC: Good for eyesight, hair growth, guarding against colds, wound healing and a healthy sex life. Also fortifies the immune system. If you take too much Zinc, you will block the absorption of another vital nutrient, copper.

SELENIUM: An essential mineral that may help you to avoid cancer in later life, and which works with a **zinc** supplement.

HYDERGINE: To keep your memory on the job, hydergine 4, 5 mg has been found to be helpful—put under your tongue and allow it to dissolve. This is available on prescription.

BORON: an essential mineral for healthy bones and vital for people with inflammatory conditions such as arthritis.

CARNOSINE: regenerates ageing cells and skin, improves muscle tone and reduces arterial plaque.

ESSENTIAL FATTY ACIDS:
Omega-3 is a fish oil and is the name given to polyunsaturated fatty acids which are essential to your diet.

Cod Liver Oil in capsule form (Vitamin A & D) is useful for the skin (psoriasis and eczema), for joints (arthritis), for the brain (dementia), for the retina, for inflammatory bowel disease, for the regulation of all biological functions, including those of the cardiovascular, reproductive, and immune and nervous system (depression).

FUEL FOR YOUR BODY: Liquids and Food

To help cleanse your body from toxins, drink a minimum of 1 litre of water per day. Drink BEFORE meals and NOT during them as this can lead to Arthritis. Most of the food we eat contains water.

PERCENTAGE OF WATER IN FOODS:

cottage cheese	74%	veal	71%
eggs	74%	beef	67%
chicken	61%	lamb	66%
cod	87%	pork	50%
tuna	57%	oyster	87%
most vegetables	90%	most fruits	80%

For better digestion and absorption of proteins and nutrients, CHEW your food until it is reduced to a paste before swallowing it.

DIGESTIVE SYSTEM

It extracts the goodness of what you eat and rejects what must be eliminated daily.

Observe the watchword "KYBO"—a name given to a racehorse—for "Keep Your Bowels Open". If having difficulties, a tea made of cherry stems; Figs or prunes can be of help. Your chemist can recommend a good laxative.

HEALTHY EATING & WEIGHT PROBLEMS

Select what you put in your mouth and you can choose your weight.

> The Victorians believed it was good to leave the table with a feeling that one would like to start all over again.

Stop thinking "diet" and start thinking "eating more healthily".

And to make a life-long change in your diet, cut down starchy and sugary foods (refined carbohydrates, artificial sweeteners and sweets, fried and fast foods) and reduce table salt. Avoid alcohol, coffee, full-fat cheeses and butter; and take minimum amounts of sugar and sweets and eat a varied diet that contains plenty of fibres (fresh fruit and vegetables) and eat one portion of quality protein a day such as fish, eggs, chicken and filets of beef.

Learn to maintain healthy habits: ALWAYS eat breakfast!
Drink lots of water or herbal teas between meals. Eat a light supper. Do not smoke. Take exercises.

If you are still finding it hard to lose weight despite eating healthy and exercising, consult a qualified medical practitioner.

You may be emotionally upset, stressed or have an under-active thyroid, a chronic food intolerance that is causing water retention, or an overloaded liver that's allowing toxins to accumulate, which your body may be storing away in fat cells.

CRAMP

For relief, take Magnesium, Potassium and Selenium and try to drink at least 1 litre of water a day.

GASTRO-ENTERITIS

Is an infection but can also be caused by drinking CONTAMINATED WATER. First of all, go to bed and rest. Drink at least one litre of bottled water—it is the safest. Then it is advisable to eat boiled rice, steamed carrots and bananas for a day or two only—don't eat meat, fresh fruits or vegetables or sweets.

KIDNEY STONES

An excess of URIC ACID causes kidney stones. Suggested remedies are NIACIN [Vitamin B3], Vitamin C in the form of Sodium Ascorbate. Baking Soda [Sodium Bicarbonate] may help.

INFLUENZA AND THE COMMON COLD

Both these are viral infections. Vitamin C can reduce their symptoms. **A dose of up to 1 gram vitamin C EFFERVESCENT should be taken first thing in the morning on an empty stomach** at the start of the symptoms, then repeated as required.

Selenium (up to 300 micrograms daily) is the body's greatest detoxifier. Before taking these doses, <u>consult your health authority.</u>

PROSTATE

The prostate is a temperamental but essential organ. When one is busy on the telephone, it demands one go in the bathroom, but on other occasions when one wishes otherwise, it shuts down.

General Research has resulted in proposing the berries of the Saw Palmetto plant, which are available in capsule form 400 mg, and the root of stinging nettle 240 mg. This should be taken twice a day.

The Saw Palmetto plant grows in Florida and is used as one of the treatments for benign enlarged prostate. The clinical benefits are the following: reduction of nocturnal urinary urgency by relaxing the bladder and sphincter muscles, increasing urinary flow rate, and reducing both the residual volume in the bladder and uncomfortable urination symptoms.

In addition to Saw Palmetto's supplement, two large studies published in 2000 showed that men who had a diet high in cruciferous vegetables (broccoli, cauliflower, cabbage, kale, Brussels sprouts) had a statistically significant reduction in the risk of prostate cancer.

It is very important to empty your bladder completely—you must be patient for several minutes—because otherwise an infection may start.

YOUR IMMUNE SYSTEM

To enable your immune system to protect you from viruses, diseases, deadly microbes all around you, and within you, **your body must be in 'CHEMICAL NEUTRAL'.** When your body is out of balance chemically cancer and other diseases can start.

This was stated by Dr. Revici of Hungary and Dr. Burns when he was the Doctor for the Newport Hospital in Rhode Island, United States.

To supervise the chemical balance of your body use LITMUS paper on your urine to verify that your body is in chemical neutral, **not too alkaline or too acid.**

If the Litmus paper turns <u>green</u>, your body may be too **alkaline.** You must bring your body back to chemical neutral with anti-histamine or Elixir of Benadryl. The neutral colour is roughly that of the Litmus paper.

If the Litmus paper turns <u>deep pink</u>, your body may be too acid. Your **acidity** level must be reduced to chemical neutral by taking bicarbonate of soda.

Do not eat big meals or drink alcohol when physically and mentally tired because your body may not be able to digest them. This will cause TOXICITY in your body and may give you a sick headache.

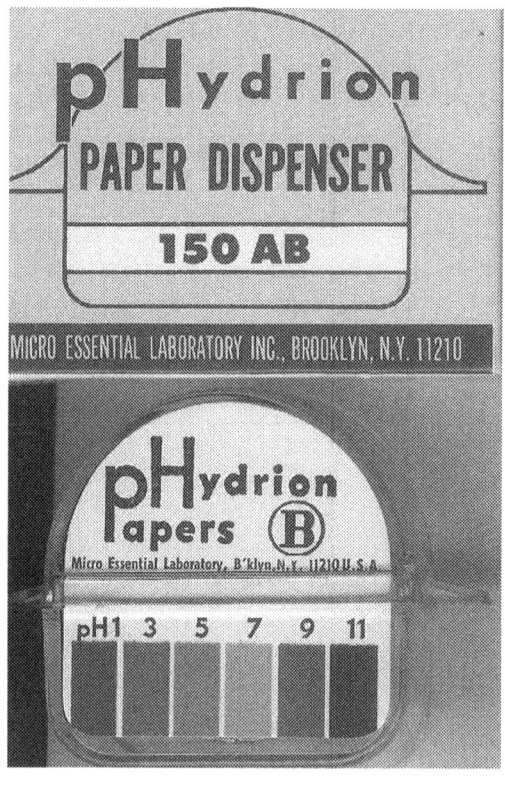

Litmus paper in a plastic dispenser can be obtained at your local pharmacy or chemist.

For further information, contact:

www.microessentiallab.com

The pH scale is from 0–14

Healthy = 7.35–7.45

> YOUR BODY MUST BE KEPT IN CHEMICAL NEUTRAL AT ALL TIMES: TOXINS ARE POISONOUS.

Are You Eating Enough Alkaline Foods to Maintain Vital Health?

The chart below categorizes a food as either acidic or alkaline based on the effect consumption of the food has on urine pH. For example, if a food tends to increase the acidity of urine after it is ingested, it is classified as an acid forming food.

Conversely, if a food increases the alkalinity of urine after it has been ingested, it is classified as an alkaline forming food. The effect foods have on urine pH may be quite different from the pH of the foods themselves. For example, orange juice is a highly acidic food due to its high citrus acid content, but after being metabolized it will cause urine to become alkaline.

Allergic reactions and other forms of stress tend to produce acids in the body. The presence of high acidity indicates that more of your foods should be selected from the alkalizing group.

> You are unique, but for most people,
> the ideal diet is 75 percent alkalizing
> and 25 percent acidifying
> foods by volume.

ALKALIZING FOODS

VEGETABLES
Garlic
Asparagus
Fermented Veggies
Watercress
Beets
Broccoli
Brussel sprouts
Cabbage
Carrot
Cauliflower
Celery
Chard
Chlorella
Collard Greens
Cucumber
Dandelion greens
Eggplant
Kale
Kohlrabi
Lettuce
Mushrooms
Mustard Greens
Dulce
Dandelions
Edible Flowers
Onions
Parsnips (high glycemic)
Peas
Peppers
Pumpkin
Rutabaga
Sea Veggies
Spinach
Sprouts
Squashes
Alfalfa
Barley & Wheat Grass
Wild Greens
Nightshade Veggies

**ALKALIZING
MINERALS**
Calcium: pH 12
Cesium: pH 14
Magnesium: pH 9
Potassium: pH 14
Sodium: pH 14

FRUITS
Apple
Apricot
Avocado
Banana (high glycemic)
Cantaloupe
Cherries
Currants
Dates/Figs
Grapes
Grapefruit
Lime
Honeydew Melon
Nectarine
Orange
Lemon
Peach
Pear
Pineapple
All Berries
Tangerine
Tomato
Tropical Fruits
Watermelon

PROTEIN
Eggs
Whey Protein Powder
Cottage Cheese
Chicken Breast
Yogurt
Almonds
Chestnuts
Tofu (fermented)
Flax Seeds
Pumpkin Seeds
Tempeh (fermented)
Squash Seeds
Sunflower Seeds
Millet
Sprouted Seeds
Nuts

OTHER
Apple Cider Vinegar
Bee Pollen
Lecithin Granules
Probiotic Cultures
Green Juices
Veggies Juices
Fresh Fruit Juice
Organic Milk
(unpasteurized)
Mineral Water
Alkaline Antioxidant Water
Green Tea
Herbal Tea
Dandelion Tea
Ginseng Tea
Banchi Tea
Kombucha

SWEETENERS
Stevia

SPICES/SEASONINGS
Cinnamon
Curry
Ginger
Mustard
Chili Pepper
Sea Salt
Miso
Tamari
All Herbs

ORIENTAL VEGETABLES
Maitake
Daikon
Dandelion Root
Shitake
Kombu
Reishi
Nori
Umeboshi
Wakame
Sea Veggies

ACIDIFYING FOODS

FATS & OILS
Avocado Oil
Canola Oil
Corn Oil
Hemp Seed Oil
Flax Oil
Lard
Olive Oil
Safflower Oil
Sesame Oil
Sunflower Oil

FRUITS
Cranberries
Blueberries
Canned or Glazed Fruits
Currants

GRAINS
Rice Cakes
Wheat Cakes
Amaranth
Barley
Buckwheat
Corn
Oats (rolled)
Quinoi
Rice (all)
Rye
Spelt
Kamut
Wheat
Hemp Seed Flour

DAIRY
Cheese, Cow
Cheese, Goat
Cheese, Processed
Cheese, Sheep
Milk
Butter

NUTS & BUTTERS
Cashews
Brazil Nuts
Peanuts
Peanut Butter
Pecans
Tahini
Walnuts

ANIMAL PROTEIN
Beef
Carp
Clams
Fish
Lamb
Lobster
Mussels
Oyster
Pork
Rabbit
Salmon
Shrimp
Scallops
Tuna
Turkey
Venison

PASTA (WHITE)
Noodles
Macaroni
Spaghetti

OTHER
Distilled Vinegar
Wheat Germ
Potatoes

DRUGS & CHEMICALS
Chemicals
Drugs, Medicinal
Drugs, Psychedelic
Pesticides
Herbicides

ALCOHOL
Beer
Spirits
Hard Liquor
Wine

BEANS & LEGUMES
Black Beans
Chick Peas
Green Peas
Kidney Beans
Lentils
Lima Beans
Pinto Beans
Red Beans
Soy Beans
Soy Milk
White Beans
Rice Milk
Almond Milk

ACIDIFYING JUNK FOOD
Beer: pH 2.5
Coca-Cola: pH 2
Coffee: pH 4

OXIDATION and AGEING

Ageing is principally caused by oxidation, a process of BIO-CHEMICAL DECAY. Changing a few HABITS can slow down this degradation and reduce the risks of premature illness and death by eliminating TOXICITY.

Everyone has the responsibility and the opportunity to cleanse the body of damaging toxins and in doing so, to IMPROVE THE QUALITY OF LIFE and to extend it. If the right measures are taken, you can look and feel YOUNGER.

LUNGS

When you begin to experience tiredness in your limbs or become forgetful, the cause of this may be either that your lungs are NOT PRODUCING ENOUGH OXYGEN or that ARTERIES ARE BLOCKED. It is very important to do deep breathing exercises every day—it will increase your vitality.

OXYGEN

Oxygen is essential to life and is extracted by your lungs from the air you breathe.

POLLUTION of the air from the burning of fossil fuels and from smoking is dangerous, making it more difficult for the lungs to extract sufficient oxygen.

NOTE: A minimum of 80% OF OXYGEN must be in your BLOOD AT ALL TIMES.

It is essential that your blood, which is the oxygen carrier, is able to circulate at least **80% of oxygen** to your brain and other parts of your body such as your immune system, digestive and reproductive organs. You can have the oxygen percentage in your blood measured by lung specialist doctors.

SLEEP

No matter where, no matter who, Oxygen from fresh, <u>pure air</u> is essential for everyone to attain a relaxed sleep.
<u>Before lying down, do deep breathing raising your arms to open your chest and lungs.</u>

If you share your bedroom with another person—make sure you sleep with a window open. It's not a good idea to share your bedroom with pets, cats or many animals—they rob you available oxygen.

STRESS

Stress is a major cause of accelerated ageing. Your best strategy for staying younger longer is to be calm and be positive.
Straight thinking is the greatest insurance against overwork and mental breakdown. **Stress triggers heart attacks, strokes, cancers, stomach ulcers and even Alzheimer's.**

Learn what your limits are and do not push yourself beyond them.

> Do not drink coffee or eat sugary snacks (chocolate bars) to keep you going when stressed.

CHECK YOUR BLOOD PRESSURE

Your blood pressure is a valuable indication of your health. To check this, ask your doctor or buy a simple machine at any chemist. It works with batteries and shows your pressure (normal is considered to be 14/8).

METAL POISONING AND BLOCKED ARTERIES

If you were brought up in an old house with lead water pipes, you may have lead poisoning.

> Concentration of LEAD, ALUMINIUM and MERCURY may increase as we age and can cause cancer, neurological dysfunction, memory loss, chronic fatigue, multiple sclerosis, infertility and heart disease called a stroke.

Some metals, used for certain food and drink cans and jar lids, ready-made meals in aluminium containers, lunch boxes, toothpaste tubes, deodorant, medicines or vaccines may contain **LEAD**, **ALUMINIUM** or **MERCURY**.

MERCURY poisoning can contribute to MEMORY DECLINE and INFERTILITY.

Environmental protection committees in most Western countries have issued a warning that fish from deep oceans and rivers contain levels of methyl mercury.

Mercury-based amalgam dental fillings are doing the most damage to our health. Mercury can be replaced by gold, though porcelain is safer.

When opening a can of food, transfer it immediately into a plastic or glass container, especially if the food must be kept for 2 or 3 days or longer.

Clean metal lids regularly, in particular for acidic condiments like mustard or pickles. For safety, use COOKING PANS that are copper silver-lined or heavy-duty enamelled steel.

Metal poison in arteries causes a build-up of fibrous material called PLAQUES. These trap particles from rich foods and impede the flow of blood carrying oxygen to the brain and other parts of the body—kidneys, lung and sexual organs.

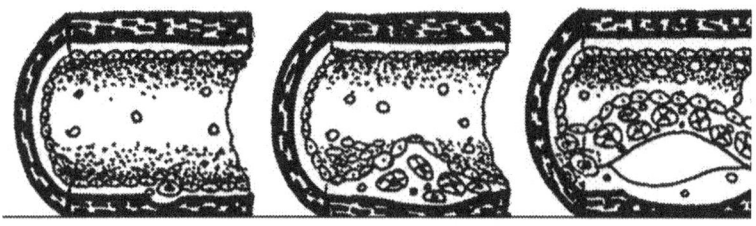

Fig. A

Healthy artery   Partly blocked   Blocked

FOR HEALTHY ARTERIES

1. Reduce bad CHOLESTEROL (foods rich in fat, sugar)
2. Stop SMOKING and reduce ALCOHOL intake
3. Drink at least 1 litre of WATER daily
4. WALK as much as you can daily

> Plaques block the arteries, and produce ARTERIOSCLERO-
> SIS. **SMOKING and HIGH BLOOD PRESSURE** are con-
> tributing factors to heart strain.

BLOOD IS INCOMPRESSIBLE.

Therefore, when arteries and veins become totally blocked, the heart is unable
to pump against the blockage.
This is in fact, a hydraulic problem—but the heart is always blamed and this is
called a "heart attack" or a stroke.

> Enhanced capillary circulation brings oxygen and nutrient-
> rich blood to the most distant of our body's cells, and carries
> away waste and carbon dioxide.

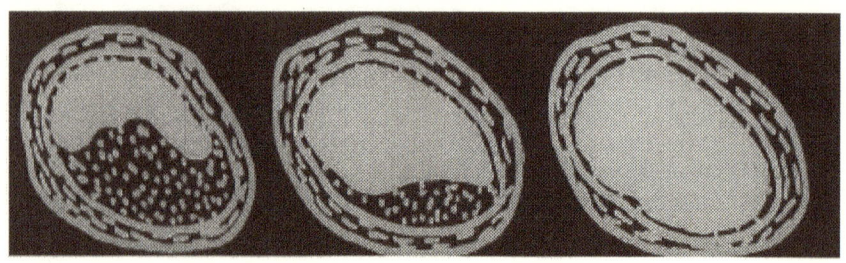

Bad   Better   Good
Fig. B—EDTA Chelation progression in arteries

BLOOD TESTS by a qualified professional laboratory will reveal if there are toxic metals such as lead, mercury, or aluminium in your arteries. To prevent them from poisoning your arteries your doctor should prescribe the following medicines which will gradually eliminate most toxins and not impede the flow of oxygen in your arteries:

E.D.T.A: Ethyl Diamine Tetra Ascetic Acid, a weak Amino Acid—related to vinegar. It has been used since 1940 for removing Lead, Mercury and Aluminium and plaque formation from arteries.

CHLORELLA: fresh water mono cellular alga which is included in E.D.T.A, contains Chlorophyll, a detoxifying and anti mutagenic component

OIL OF OREGANO: natural antiseptic, anti-fungal and aids digestion

BEAR'S or WILD GARLIC: *allium ursinum*—rich in mineral substances

CORIANDER: Vitamin C, helps the body to absorb iron and accelerates healing after surgery

PECTIN: Natural compounds in the pectin (citrus) unclog the obstructions in the blood vessels that can trigger the stroke or heart attack

HIGH DOSE PROBIOTICS: lactobacillus acidophilus, they support intestinal health

WARNING:

E.D.T.A. and other substances may and can remove IRON or other important minerals from your body—your doctor will make a blood test and tell you if you need iron or another important mineral and he will prescribe what you need.

It is advisable to take **multi mineral complex** (Calcium, Chromium, Copper, Magnesium, Selenium, Zinc, Boron and Vanadium) after meals while the oral chelators (E.D.T.A) should be taken on an empty stomach between meals (at least 3 or 4 hours between those products).

To order consult chapter on *Useful Information and Address.*

OSTEOPOROSIS (Brittle Bones)

Osteoporosis, or bone brittleness, more common in women than men, is due mainly to the diminishing production in the body of the hormone oestrogen.

Only too often, this condition leads to broken hips and cracked vertebrae.

Hormone activity in women decreases, particularly after the age of 50, and, in the past doctors advised taking supplementary oestrogen, generally in tablet form in order to prevent osteoporosis—commonly called H.R.T or Hormone Replacement Therapy (oestrogen alone or oestrogen plus progestin, artificial hormones).

Studies, concluded in 2003 and 2004, show H.R.T can produce unwanted side-effects.

Doctors have stated that testosterone may be safer in general than oestrogen.

Supplemental testosterone is needed if total testosterone is low. A blood test will confirm whether your level of testosterone is too low. Too low a level may contribute to osteoporosis.

It is known that some women continue to produce testosterone even in menopause. Loss of libido is caused by too low a level of testosterone—men should be interested as well as women.

Low levels of "free" testosterone are associated with risk of Alzeimer's. Every woman's requirements may be different; therefore, take professional advice and consult your doctor to insure that what you take is right for your case.

FOR MEN AS WELL AS WOMEN: Healthy eating, which includes plenty of organic vegetables and fruit, taking the right supplements and staying in shape (exercises and yoga) will also help maintain bone density.

Avoid phosphates in caffeine-based foods and drinks because phosphates steal calcium from your bones. Colas and many other carbonated soft drinks contain phosphoric acid. Phosphoric acid dissolves calcium—so do not touch them!

Avoid coffee and take minimum amount of sugar and sweets.

ACTION TO TAKE FOR OSTEOPOROSIS

The following supplements should be taken DAILY and ALWAYS on an empty stomach first thing in the morning.

CALCIUM, 500 mg	MAGNESIUM, 500 mg
BORON, 3 mg	VITAMIN K, 10 mg
ZINC, 15 mg	DHEA, 25 mg to 100 mg

First thing in the morning, VITAMIN C,1 g, and last thing at night, VITAMIN D, 1 tablespoon of Cod Liver Oil.

Also take 3 mg of Boron every day which is a trace mineral needed for healthy bones. Boron is necessary for the conversion of Vitamin D and helps the body to produce natural oestrogen.

Vitamin K, 10 mg per day helps keep calcium in the bones and out of the arteries; found in green leafy vegetables. Also take zinc (15 mg per day).

<u>Vitamin D is essential</u>: Take it in the D3 form of cod liver oil 400 IUs—say one tablespoon full—taken last thing at night before going to bed. It allows the body to absorb calcium and phosphorous needed for healthy bones.

DHEA (Dehydroepiandrosterone)

<u>DHEA is a vital steroid hormone and comes in capsules of 25 to 100 mg to suit varying abilities for absorption.</u>

DHEA is naturally produced in healthy, young bodies, but as the body ages DHEA levels fall.

When you are getting on in years, you may need to take 100 mg or 200 mg or more to suit your work load.

DHEA builds up body tissues. It is the most abundant steroid hormone in the body. It comes from cholesterol and can be converted in your body into oestrogen or testosterone.

> REGULAR EXERCISES INCREASE DHEA LEVELS

It is stated that DHEA helps prevent brain ageing, cancer, heart disease, and both bone and skin degeneration and protects against Alzheimer's and dementia and also boosts the immune system and improves one's mood.

A note of caution because DHEA can be metabolized into testosterone and oestrogen, DHEA use should be avoided by anyone who currently has prostate cancer or breast cancer.

DHEA is not available in many countries, to order check chapter on *Useful Information and Addresses.*

ARTHRITIS

Experts in America say about arthritis sufferers "you should NOT DRINK WITH MEALS", but a ½ hour before or 1 hour afterwards. Avoid foods such as oils with sugar, ice cream, butter substitutes, nuts and acids such as citrus fruits. These can destroy cartilage in your joints. It is important to keep your body in chemical neutral.

GLUCOSAMINE taken WITH CONDROITIN SULPHATE and BORON help lubricate and repair the cartilage in your joints.

FOR ENHANCED TREATMENT

1.   Greatly reduce coffee, alcohol, black tea, cows' milk, red meat, high-fat cheeses, fried foods, sausages, meat pies and chocolate as these are all ACID forming.

2.   Eat LEAN meat, oily fish such as mackerel, halibut, salmon and tuna, as the Omega-3 oil contained in these has good healing power. Include in your diet plenty of green vegetables: lettuce, cucumbers, squashes, carrots, asparagus and cauliflower, as well as fruit such as apples, apricots, pears, cantaloupe melons, cherries, plums, peaches and in particular, raisins, figs and prunes.

3.   Take ONE tablespoon of pure COD Liver Oil (Vitamin D) LAST THING AT NIGHT.

SEXUALITY

Another cause for imbalance can be insufficient sexual activity. It has been stated that "**HEARTY SEX**" may add years to one's life. Physical pleasure is beneficial for both men and women.

> To regenerate sexual energy, **TONICS** such as **Garlic**, which purifies the blood, **Ginseng**, which influences the hormonal balance in the pituitary-adrenal axis, and **Ginger roots**, which boosts the circulatory system and in turn produces resistance to infections, as well as **Noni juice**, can be used as mild aphrodisiacs and for repairs to the healing system.

TEETH

The teeth are for chewing and breaking down food in the mouth in order to make digestion easier.

The action of chewing with your teeth (their primary function) is the first link in the chain of digestion. The teeth should pulverise the food into a semi-liquid state for easy swallowing.

Do not "gobble" or swallow lumps of food that are not properly masticated.

The stomach's job is to digest the already well broken down food—it is not equipped with teeth—so be sure it is properly chewed up before you swallow or you risk painful indigestion.

It is said that the Victorian Prime Minister, Mr. Gladstone, chewed each mouthful 32 times before swallowing!

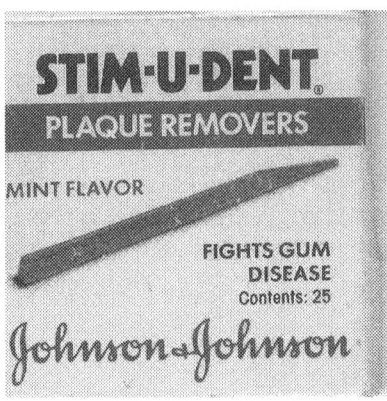

Try to clean your teeth after each meal, not just at bedtime, in order to PRE-VENT PLAQUE forming. Use a water pick, Stim-U-Dents or dental floss to dislodge all bits of food. Choose a medium hard toothbrush and toothpaste without fluoride, if possible—**never keep a toothbrush for more than 3 months.** Have three toothbrushes, one per meal.

Brush the back and front of your teeth, then gums and tongue to stimulate blood circulation. Do this for 5 minutes (This is one of life's best investments) and massage the gums with your fingers to ensure better circulation of blood carrying oxygen.

Put a teaspoon of PEROXIDE in warm water to rinse. If you have dentures, caps or crowns, use a pinch of SEA SALT instead for well-known antiseptic and healing benefits.

Go to a DENTIST at least twice a year to have plaque removed. When in pain, do check for ROOT DECAY. REGULAR VISITS are important as it has been proved that a decayed root canal can cause pain in other parts of your body.

SKIN CARE

A dermatologist is the correct person to ask for a suitable skin care formula because not all of them may suit you.

Remember both men and women NEED regular skin care and this may change with increasing years. Drink water and do not smoke and sunbathe too much.

The following supplements are helpful daily: Carnosine (150 mg), Vitamin C (1 gram), Vitamin A (in the form of beta-carotene 30 mg), Vitamin E (200 IUs), Zinc (10 mg), Selenium (150 mg) and Essential Fats, Omega-3s.

EARS AND HEARING

Ability to hear is largely governed by the physical condition of your body. It is vital that your immune system be maintained in the <u>highest</u> possible condition.

When you wash and bathe, be careful to dry your ears with a soft cloth or towel—cleanliness is very important.
Noises in the ears (**Tinnitus**) may be alleviated by taking Ginkgo Biloba leaves; used by the Chinese for more than a 1000 years.

One's hearing ability will be affected by any brief exposures to loud noises on a regular basis such as heavy machinery in some factories, gunshots, jet engines or any other very loud and sudden noises. But even worse, listening to loudly amplified noises called "Pop" music.

If you are subjected to such noises you can block your ears. Seriously, if you attend a "Pop" concert you will be well advised to provide yourself with earplugs. It is unlikely that the damage caused by overstressing your hearing mechanism can be recovered.

SINUS PROBLEMS

Sinus problems are usually caused by an allergy from pollen, dust and/or mildew.

First thing in the morning, clean your nose with warm salt water before brushing your teeth.

Allergic reactions tend to produce acids in the body. The presence of high acidity indicates that more of your foods should be selected from the alkalizing group.

Check your immune system and consult your doctor for the best suitable treatment.

PART TWO: MASSAGES AND PHYSICAL EXERCISES TO IMPROVE YOUR HEALTH

EYES

GLAUCOMA

Eyesight deterioration with age is very difficult to detect. LUTEIN and ZEAXANTHIN can improve pigment density in the retina and help reduce MACULAR DEGENERATION. Zeaxanthin is found in green leafy vegetables, peaches and mangoes. BILBERRY extract is also effective.

TENSION AND STRAIN can cause medical difficulties, such as POOR VISION. Sight problems are often accompanied by patterns of muscle tension. For example, those who suffer MYOPIA, tend to have pressure in the forehead, jaw, neck, shoulders, arms, lower back and even in the calves or legs.

MACULAR DEGENERATION. This is a most serious defect. Be sure and ask your Eye Doctor to tell you what action you should take NOW, to avoid the disability of macular degeneration which destroys the nerve connections to the brain.

PROTECTION AGAINST BRIGHT SUNLIGHT

Wear dark glasses that filter INFRARED, YELLOW and ULTRAVIOLET rays. Do not stare at the sun and NEVER look at it during an eclipse. It can burn your retina.

EYE MASSAGE AND EXERCISES

Everyone, especially children, should do eye exercises every morning. With this in mind, here are some suggestions for various massage points that may help to improve your vision naturally. The following instructions are for self-massage.

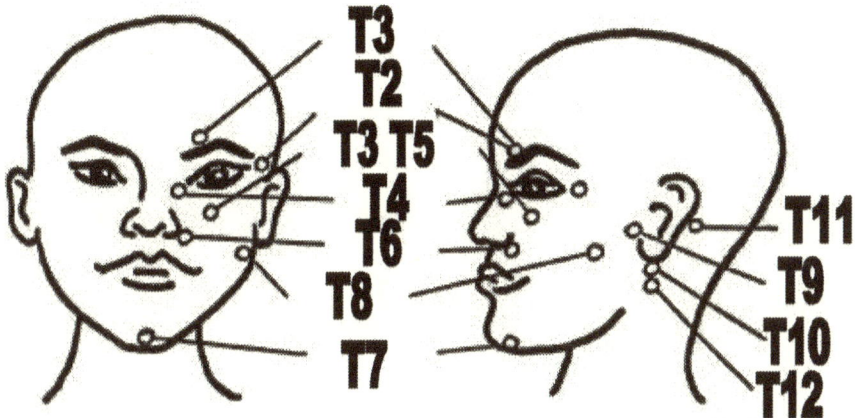

Fig. A
Start by washing your hands and make sure your fingers are warm.

<u>Refer to the numbers on the diagram.</u>
- To strengthen these muscles, begin by closing both eyes tightly and keep them shut for 10-15 seconds.
- Then open your eyes wide and make a great effort to stretch your face raising your eyebrows [T3] as high as possible.
- Place your fingers on your chin [T7] and gently move them upwards each side of your jaw to underneath and behind your ears [T12]. Use a good massage skin cream.
- Open your jaws fully, then close them and repeat 5 times. Massage gently but firmly the part under your ears [T12]
- Move from there to the bridge of your nose and downwards across the top of your cheek bones [T5] to your ears [T8 and T12].
- Back to the bridge of your nose [T4]—squeeze it gently then move outwards on to your right eyebrow, form a curve under the right eye on top of the cheekbones then to the bridge of your nose, then to the left eyebrow followed by   the same pressure under the left eye on top of the

cheekbones up the bridge of the nose and to the right eyebrow, followed by long strokes right up to your ears.
- Do this several times and stretch your eyebrows and work your fingers in an oval movement.

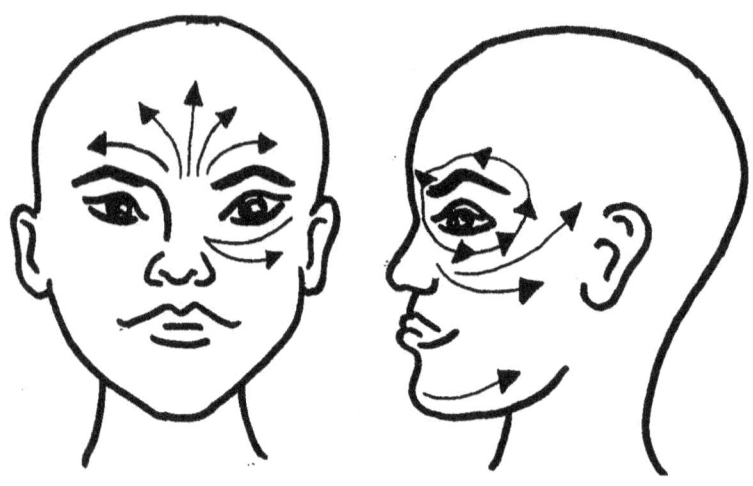

Fig. B
- Massage gently but firmly under your ears. From there, move to the bridge of your nose, then downwards across the top of your cheekbones. Go back to your ears, then the NOSE BRIDGE (squeezing it gently).
- Circle the bone around the EYE SOCKET. Do this for each side. Finish long strokes towards your ears. Repeat several times.
- Move up and across your forehead with long and firm finger movements. Keep at it for several minutes without interruption.

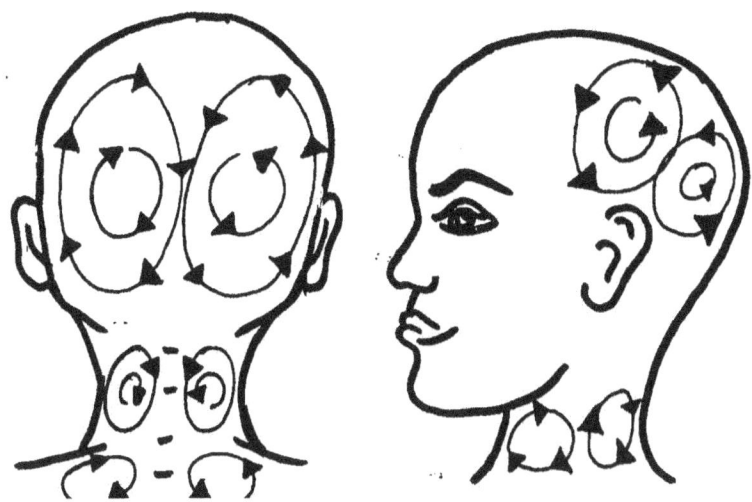

Fig. C
- Also massage the side and the back of your head and neck and notice *HOW MUCH BETTER YOU FEEL!*

Working the eye muscles everyday improves vision and STRENGTH, which may DELAY DETERIORATION later in life.

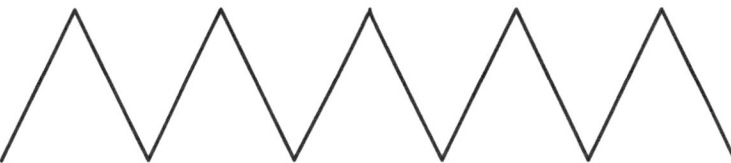

Fig. D—Look above, and with both your eyes, follow the peaks and valleys. Blink several times.

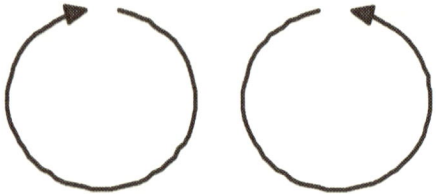

Fig. E—Rotate your eyes slowly, one at a time and then together. Repeat 10 times. Blink several times.

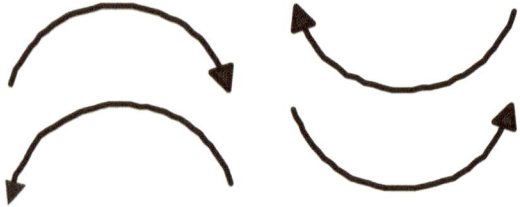

Fig. F—Follow each curve without moving your head. Go as far as possible to each corner of your eyes. Blink several times.

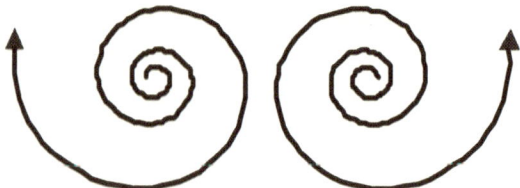

Fig. G—Follow the spirals to the left and to the right. <u>Blink again.</u>

The following vitamins, minerals and supplements are being taken with advantage by people suffering from diminished vision acuity: Zinc, Beta Carotene, Zeaxantin, Gingko Biloba, Bilberry, Selenium, Vitamin E, Lutein and Macula Plus.

NECK

SELF-MASSAGE

To massage the back of your neck, apply a few drops of Pure Oil Essences and gently rub with your fingertips. For example, to relax, select Lavender. To stimulate, use Ylang-Ylang.

1. Turn your head to the right and with your left fingers, start massaging behind the ear.

2. Move towards the top of your spine at the base of your neck, massaging, stroking and tapping gently until the muscles are softened.

3. Do the same with the other side.

FINISH WITH HEAD MOVEMENTS:

4. Start with your head straight. Lean forward. Go back straight. Lean backwards. Do it twice.

5. From the straight position, turn your head to the right as far as you can. Do it twice on each side.

6. From the straight position, lean your head on one side, getting your ear close to your shoulder. Do this twice on each side.
If you are lucky you may have a kind friend who will assist you by doing this massage for you!

SPINE

To maintain a good POSTURE and avoid a bad back in later life, use all types of support, such as a lower back cushion in your car, the right pillow and mattress to sleep on and the right chair to work in. Keeping your spine aligned and straight can be achieved with YOGA and STRETCHING movements.

MUSCLES on both sides of the top of the spine—at the base of the skull—**NEED TO BE MASSAGED** TO REDUCE TENSION AND STRESS. This could have POSITIVE EFFECTS on your EMOTIONS, therefore your well-being and that of others.

EXERCISES

LEGS AND STOMACH

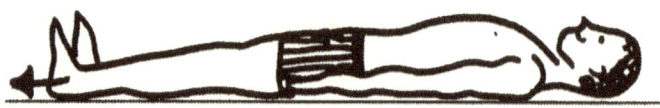

Fig. I—Lie on your back, flat on the floor on a bath towel. Stretch first one leg as far as possible; keep both heels on the floor. Relax, and then stretch the other leg. Relax.

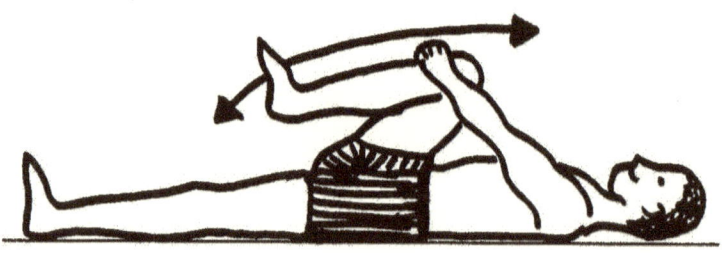

Fig. II—Next, pull up one knee as close to your stomach as possible, then the other and wriggle your toes up and down as much as you can. Repeat 4 times. With your legs bent and knees together, roll to the right and then to the left, as far as possible, keeping your body flat on the floor.

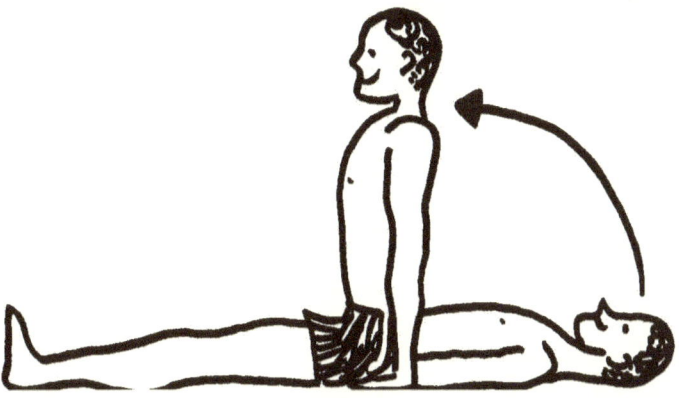

Fig. III—Keeping both legs straight on the floor, raise your torso up, keeping it straight. Then lower it slowly. Relax. Repeat several times.

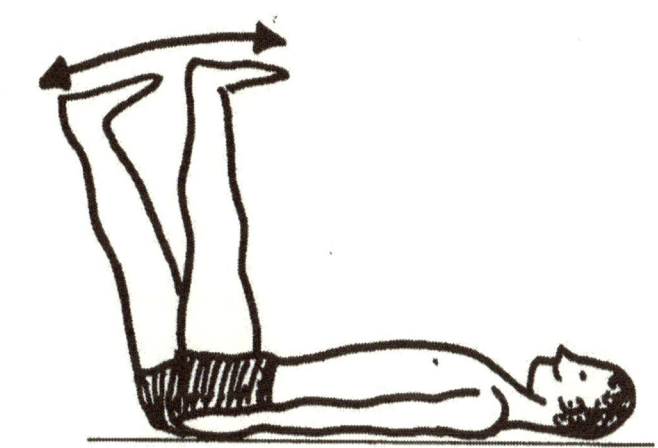

Fig. IV—Lie flat on your back, raise both legs together until they are straight up. Spread your legs keeping them straight, as wide as you can. Now bring both legs to the vertical position, and then cross over your legs back and forth several times.

ARMS AND SHOULDERS

Lie on your stomach. Put your hands flat on the floor right under your shoulders. Keep your body rigid and push yourself up. Lower your body and repeat several times. (Men only)

NECK EXERCISES

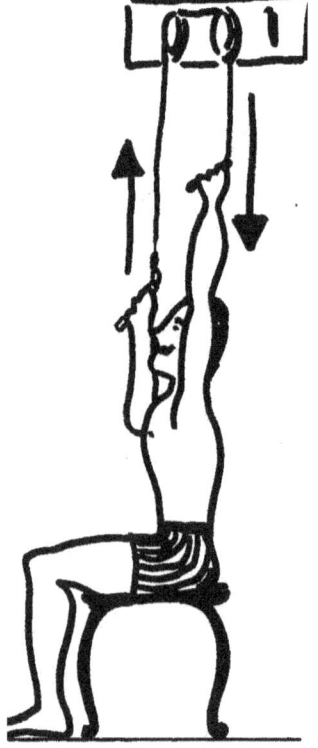

Sit straight on a stool or chair. Hold your head back as far as you can, then turn it from side to side 50 times.

Secure 2 pulleys, about 10 cm or 3 inches—whatever is available—in diameter, to the side of a beam. Place them about 30 cm or 12 inches apart. Loop a strong cord over the pulleys with both ends hanging down. Tie a big knot at each end.

Sit on a chair or stool under the pulleys. Hold the knotted end with your outstretched hand. Take the other end at about head height and tie a large knot at that point.

Fig. V—

Then sitting straight up, tilt your head back as far as possible, pull down the up stretched arm, and swing your head at the same time until the other arm is fully up stretched. Then pull down the stretched arm, swing your head and repeat 50 times.

If it isn't possible to use the pulleys and rope, sit on a chair or stool and tilt your head back as far as possible, then swing your head from side to side. Turn your head to the left, forward and downwards, then over to the right, moving it upwards and backwards in a semi-rotating motion. Repeat 10 times.

Don't be alarmed if you hear a creaking noise—this calls for neck exercises—and now repeat the same movement from right to left 10 times. Try to do these exercises every day.

PELVIC FLOOR MUSCLES

Exercising regularly prevents erectile disorders and improves sexual perform-ance: strength and endurance.

Pelvic floor exercises should become a part of every man's fitness regime health experts say: they extend and improve your sex life performance.

To strengthen your pelvic muscles and avoid INCONTINENCE, contract your buttocks as you sit or stand, anywhere, anytime, with feet apart. Maximize your time standing in line or driving, to do these exercises.

Squeeze, and then relax your anal muscles 15 times. Do this as many times as you can everyday and when walking or lying down. At first, you may find your-self squeezing your stomach and thigh muscles but within a few days, you acquire the coordination to squeeze only the pelvic muscles.

This is also good advice for women after childbirth and those who are getting on a bit.

EXERCISES IN THE SWIMMING POOL

Swimming is a great exercise so if and when you have access to a swimming pool, exercise your muscles simply by pushing against the water. For example:

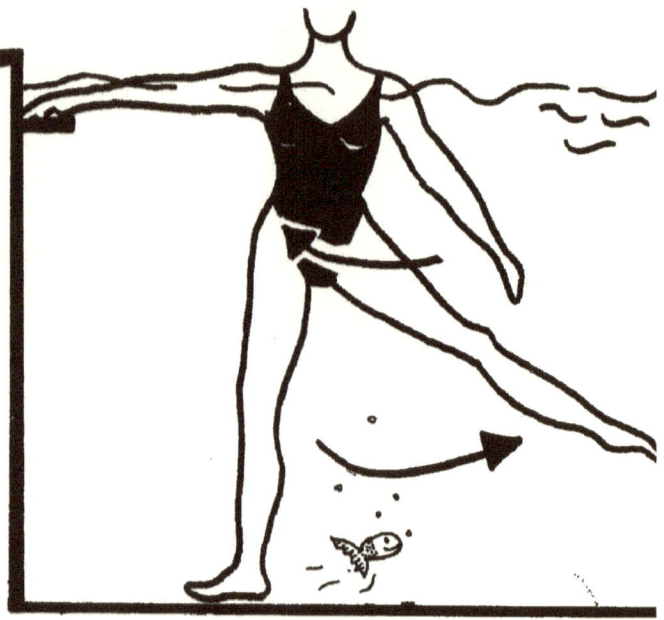

Fig. I

1. Stand with the water up to your neck. Holding on to the side of the pool, swing the right leg as high as you can to the right while pushing the right hand in the opposite direction. Do at least 6 times with each side.

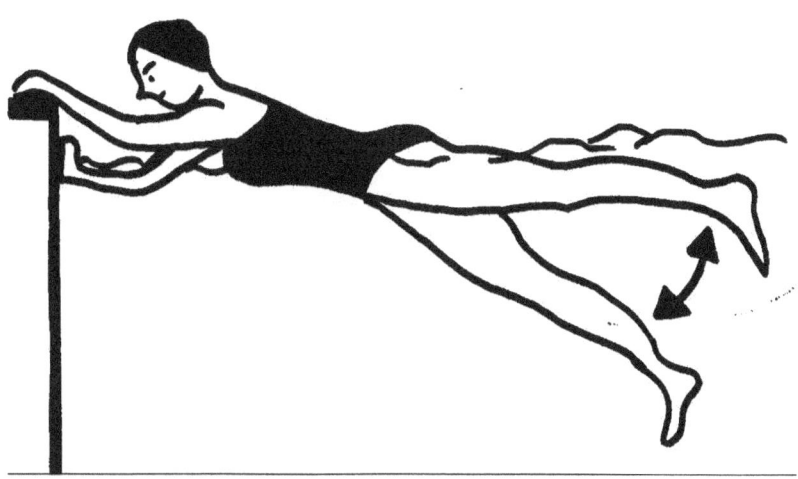

Fig. II

2. Facing the side of the pool, hold on to the side. Raise your whole body behind you to the level of the water. Kick your legs up and down, as in dog paddle. You can do this with your knees bent or your legs straight. Do this for 5 minutes.

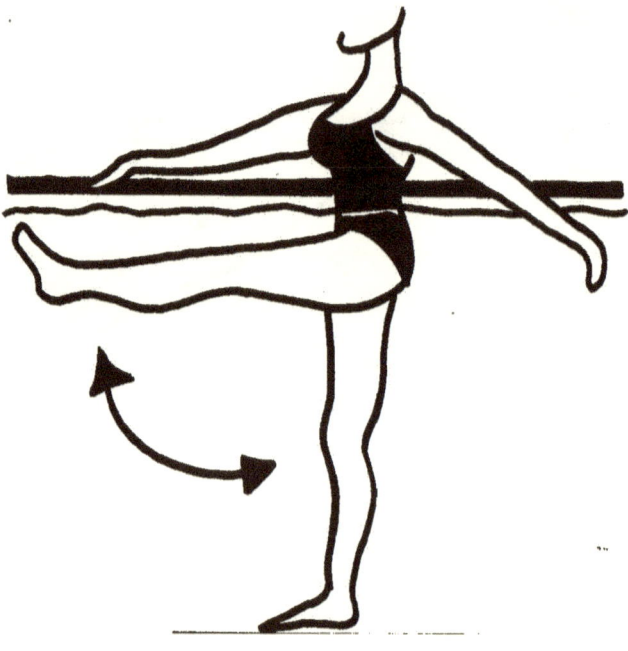

Fig. III

3. Stand sideways to the pool and swing your leg forwards and backwards, reaching as high as you can.

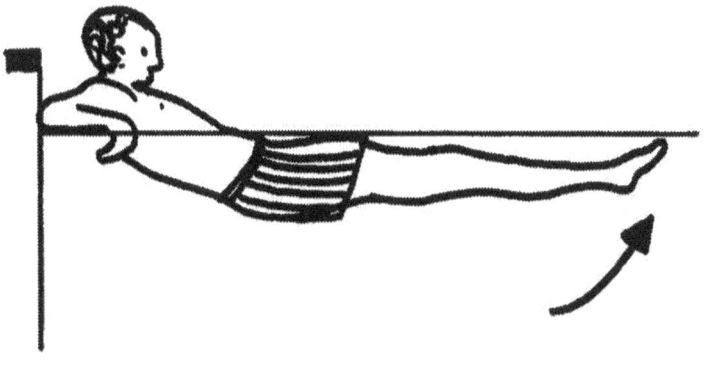

Fig. IV

4. With your back to the side of the pool, hold onto the sides with your arms outstretched. Lift both legs as high as you can in front of you. Kick up and down for 5 minutes.

Other exercises will suggest themselves to you when you are in the water. They are more effective and easier to execute than on dry land because of the weightlessness.

BODY NETWORK—MERIDIANS

The word MERIDIAN instantly brings to mind "Greenwich" and the 0° Degree of Longitude that runs from the North Pole to the South Pole through the Greenwich Observatory—built in the reign of Charles II in the 17th century—. All distances from that Greenwich MERIDIAN are measured East or West of it in degrees.

Many thousand of years ago, the Chinese used MERIDIANS to define invisible PATHWAYS that form the WEB NETWORK of your body's nervous system.

These pathways—they are not blood vessels—connect all cells and organs by going through them, linking the body's interior with its many surface points, from top to toe.

Meridian massage is an approach to therapeutic bodywork based on the manual stimulation of the body's Meridian system—it can do wonders to the network of your vital energy channels.

YOUR BODY'S WONDERFUL WORKING SYSTEMS DO NEED REGULAR ON-GOING MAINTENANCE—IN ADDITION TO FUEL (FOOD AND WATER)—TO KEEP WORKING WELL.

MERIDIAN DIAGRAMS

BLADDER PATHWAY

As an example of how channels connect different organs, the bladder pathway starts in the eyes, goes up the forehead to the top of the head, down the back of the neck, the spine, through the bladder and continues all the way to the feet via the buttocks and the legs. (Fig. I)

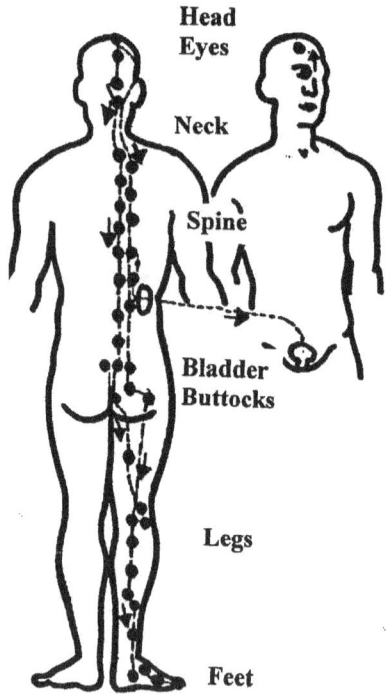

Fig. I—Bladder Pathway

The bladder is responsible for storing and excreting the urinary waste fluids passed down from the kidneys. As an organ the bladder has only this function, but as an energy system the bladder is intimately related to the functions and balance of the autonomous nervous system. If you stimulate the flow of energy along the spinal branches of the bladder meridian you directly influence the nervous system which regulates all the body's basic vital functions.

KIDNEY PATHWAY

It is known as the body's most important reservoir of essential energy "root of life". It is also the major indicator of health and immunity.

The kidneys themselves are responsible for filtering waste metabolites from the blood and moving them onwards to the bladder for excretion in urine. Along with the large intestine, the kidneys control the balance of fluids in the body.

In addition they regulate the body's ACID—ALKALINE BALANCE (pH) by selectively filtering out or retaining various minerals.

According to most sources the kidney meridian has a complex series of trajectories, both internal and external flow of the kidney channels.

LARGE INTESTINE PATHWAY

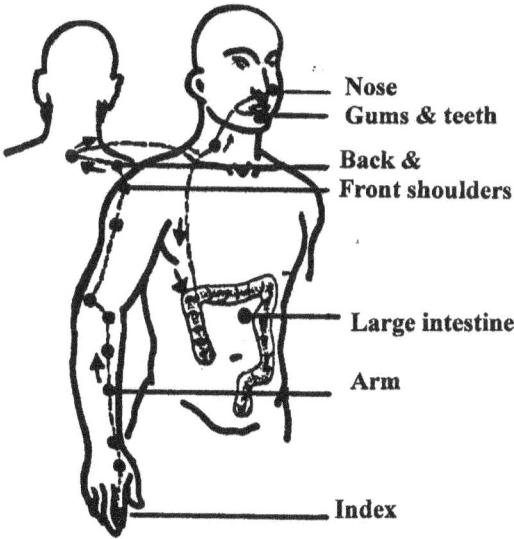

Fig. II—Large Intestine Pathway

For the LARGE INTESTINE, another pathway starts in both index fingers, goes up the arms to split like a fork at the shoulders towards the back and the front of the body, goes to the intestine and back up to end near the teeth, gum and nose.

The large intestine controls the transformation of the digestive wastes from liquid to solid state and transports the solids onwards and outwards for excretion through the rectum.
It plays a major role in the balance and purity of bodily fluids and assists the lungs in controlling the skin's pores and perspiration.

LUNGS PATHWAY

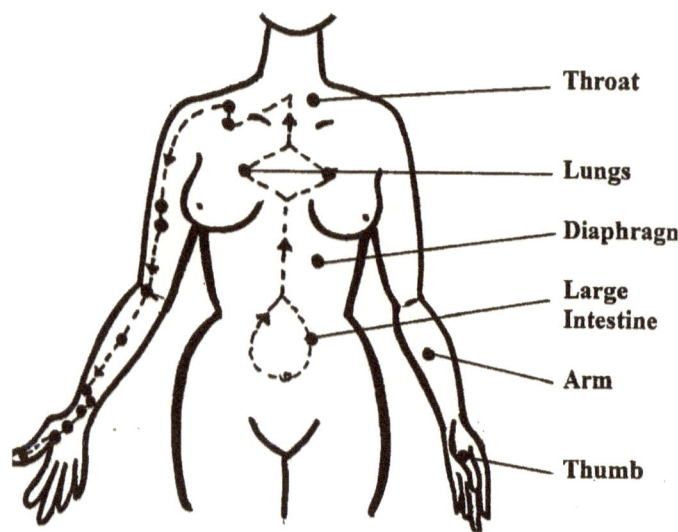

Fig. III—Lungs Pathway

And for the energy needed by the LUNGS, a pathway links the arms all the way to the tip of each thumb.

The lungs control breath and energy and assist the heart with the circulation of blood. There is an intimate relationship between regular breathing and your pulse. Breathing controls cellular respiration and shallow irregular breathing is therefore a major cause of low vitality and insufficient metabolism.

CONCLUSION

It is hoped that these notes based on actual experiences over more than 100 years in fact, will be of help.

As stated in the introduction they must not take precedence over the views of your own physician or health adviser.

Asculapius says:

"Life is NOT like a gramophone record or CD…"
I'd like that melody over again and re-play it."

If valuable minutes are misused,
you can NEVER GET THEM BACK so THINK—
and get them RIGHT THE FIRST TIME!

YOU CANNOT HAVE YOUR TIME OVER AGAIN!

"IT IS LATER THAN YOU THINK", a beautiful anonymous poem about life and time; the author has adapted the poem and has added the following closing lines:

The Oceans Await you—
Don't forget your vitamins.

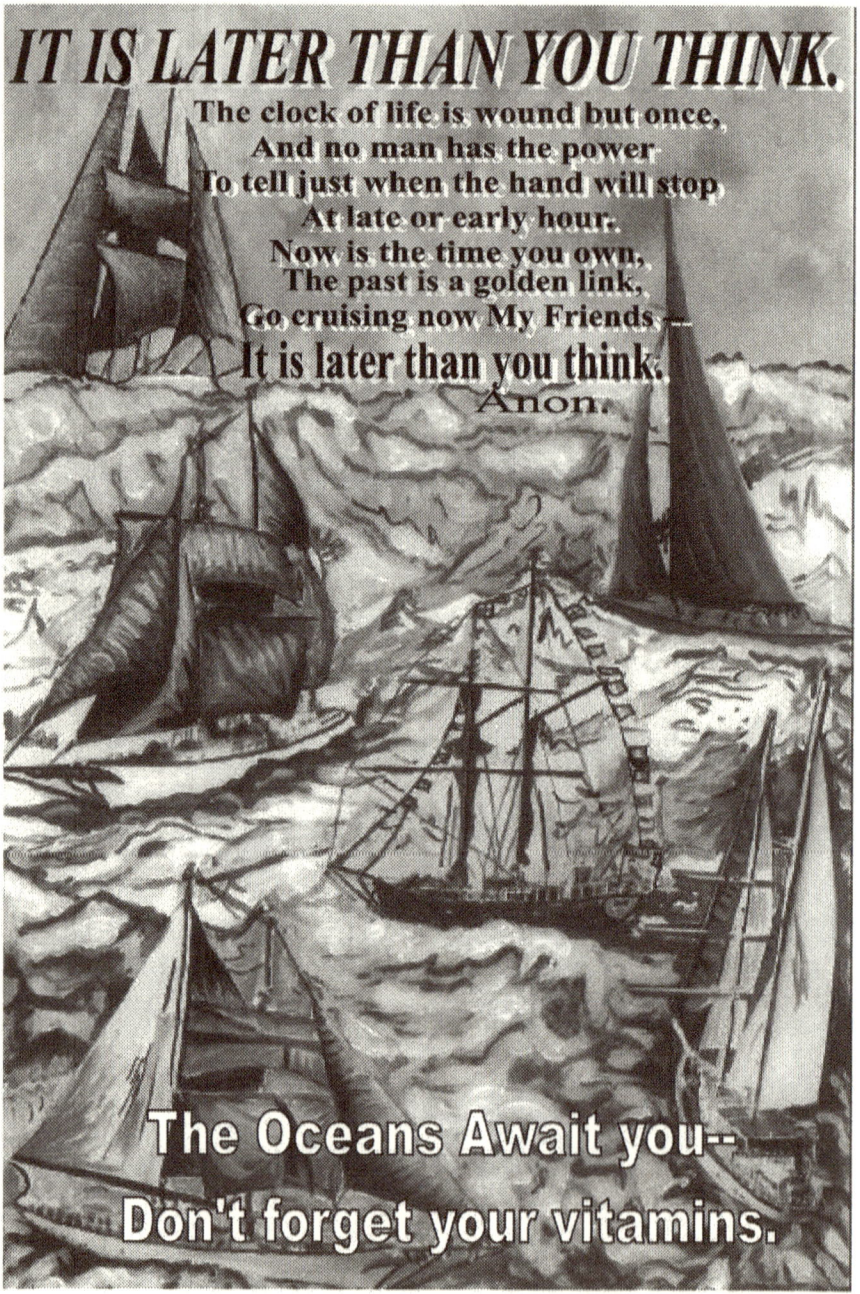

IT IS LATER THAN YOU THINK.

The clock of life is wound but once,
And no man has the power
To tell just when the hand will stop,
At late or early hour.
Now is the time you own,
The past is a golden link,
Go cruising now My Friends --
It is later than you think.

Anon.

The Oceans Await you--
Don't forget your vitamins.

Useful Information and Addresses

E.D.T.A. and other supplements
For information on E.D.T.A. Chelation:
American College for Advancement in Medicine
23121 Verdugo Dr., St 204, Laguna Hills, CA, 92653, USA, Fax: 949—455 9679
For purchasing E.D.T.A., contact SMARTCITY S.A.
B.P 3015—L—1030 Luxembourg—Grand Duché de Luxembourg, Tel: 0800 666 742 (free call)
www.supersmart.com

DHEA
The Life Extension Foundation on www.lef.org

LITMUS PAPER from Micro Essential Laboratory
www.microessentiallab.com

OSTEOPATHY
This can solve the problem at the root, it's amazing how many people have skeletal pain. An osteopath can give you help at the spot. Practitioners use manipulation, massage and stretching techniques. Always make sure the osteopath is serious and has a recognized degree.
www.osteopathy.org.uk

YOGA
Yoga teaches relaxation and breathing techniques, together with gentle stretching exercises, which help your body to remain supple forever.

THERMOSOLAR® NON-IMAGING OPTICS AT WORK

THERMOSOLAR® converts light from Non-Imaging Optics to high temperatures to pre-heat cold water.

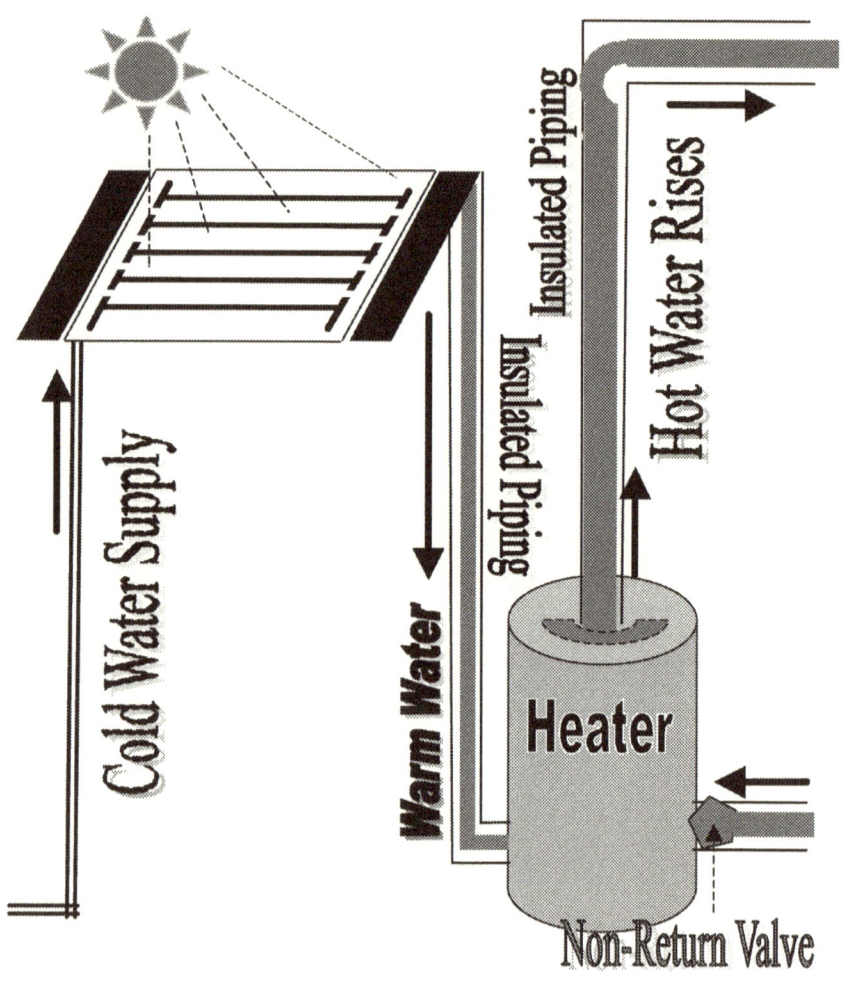

INSTANT HOT WATER is available thanks to the Thermosyphon Principle, a natural phenomenon. This will eliminate having to draw off cold water from the hot tap to get to Hot Water-this avoids wasting water.

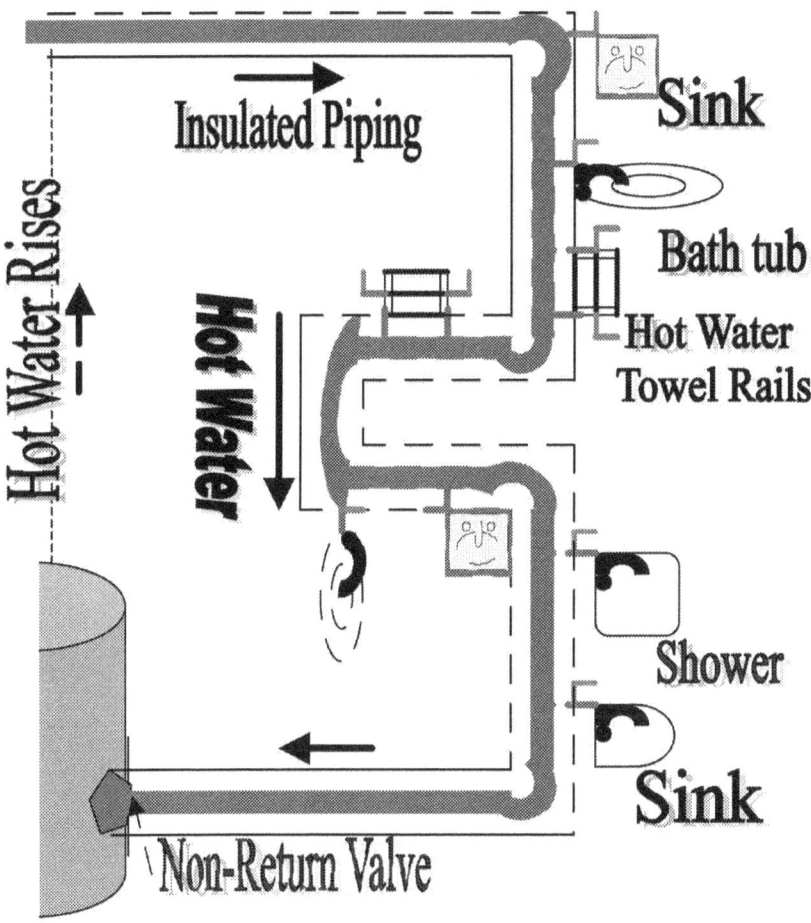

THERMOSYPHON PRINCIPLE CAN SAVE FRESH WATER

INSTANT HOT WATER is available from your boiler or water heater thanks to the Thermosyphon Principle. This eliminates having to draw off cold water from the hot tap to get to the Hot Water. Heat rises. No pump is needed.

Hot water from the boiler or water heater is carried in insulated piping from the boiler to the top of the house where Hot Water circulates down to a non-return valve on the cold side of the boiler. From this insulated return pipe, instant Hot Water is available for shower, basin or baths and hot water towel rails on all floors in the house.

To reduce the cost of heating the boiler we recommend that our **Non-Imaging Optical System** be used to collect free daylight energy for Thermosolar® to pre-heat cold water from the mains before it enters the boiler.

Many areas of the world face **inadequate supplies of fresh water**, but cannot afford either the high initial capital or daily operating costs of fossil-fuel-powered desalination plants.

<u>SAVE FUTURE WATER</u>
IT IS NEVER TOO LATE TO IMPROVE
THE QUALITY OF
BOTH OUR HEALTH AND OUR LIFE

Human demand on biosphere has increased and Earth's natural capital is only available for a limited number of people and for a limited period of time.

SAVE FUTURE WATER

Global fresh water use doubled from 1961 to 2001. Agricultural use grew by three quarters, industrial use more than doubled, and **domestic use** grew more than four-fold.

In rainy weather, gases combine with rain to form highly dangerous poisons called **ACID RAIN** that destroy farmlands in Denmark, fruit and vegetable orchards, flowers, plants, shrubs and trees in Continental Europe, especially in Germany and Switzerland and kills fish in lakes in Norway and Sweden.

We need to protect our river basins, wetlands and watershed ecosystems to sustain freshwater supply and eliminate the use of toxic chemicals that degrade ecosystems.

It's better to use a little more energy to heat water than waste water.

WATER IS LIFE.

SAVE OUR PLANET FROM POLLUTION

Energy, dominated by fossil fuels, was the fastest growing component between 1961 and 2001, increasing by nearly **700% over this period.**

Man's continuous burning of fossil fuels—coal, oil and liquid petroleum gas—has created an ever-thickening layer of poisonous gases, principally carbon dioxide and sulphur dioxide, which surrounds our planet's upper atmosphere because they do not dissipate into the super-stratosphere. They are constantly building up, trapping the heat from the sun and the heat reflected from the earth, and they affect <u>the planet's heat balance and upset our weather patterns.</u>

Burning coal and other fossil fuels to generate electricity has been replaced in other countries by the **conversion of coal into hydrogen gas** at the COAL MINES.

Hydrogen powered gas turbines generate electricity which is connected to the "GRID"—thus saving the cost of carrying coal 200 miles or more to be burnt in order to raise steam to drive turbines to generate electricity. This suggestion was submitted to the British government in May 1991.

74% of all electricity generated is used for space heating in Winter (28%), space cooling in Summer (26%) and 20% for heating cold water.

DAMAGE CAUSED BY POLLUTION

WWF International have contributed this

summary from the *Living Planet Report 2004*.

Terrestrial species such as Caribou, black rhinoceros, white-fronted goose, tiger, common brush-tailed possum, Cuckoo and oriental white-backed vulture declined by 30% between 1970 and 2000 and especially tropical terrestrial species, they fell about 65%.

Freshwater species such as Chum salmon, American wigeon, American and New Guinea crocodile, common sandpiper, hippopotamus, Ganges river dolphin, otter, black stilt and whooping crane declined by 50% from 1970 to 2000.

Marine Species such as Pacific cod, Hawaiian monk seal, green turtle, sea otter, brown pelican, southern elephant seal, Atlantic cod, herring, dugong, Fiordland penguin and indo-pacific humpbacked dolphin declined by 30% between 1970 and 2000.

Food, Fibre, and Timber grew by 42% between 1961 and 2001, with the largest increases in the use of fishing grounds (98%) and grazing land (186%).

CLIMATE CHANGE AND INCREASING POLLU-
TION FROM RISING CONSUMPTION
OF FOSSIL FUELS URGES
RAPID TRANSFER TO RENEWABLE ENERGIES OF WHICH
THE SUN IS THE PRIME SUPPLIER.

Daylight Energy Foundation promotes the SUN's DAYLIGHT POWER; NON-POLLUTING because it can heat cold water with no fuel costs.

74% of all electricity generated results in **POLLUTING OUR PLANET** and could—and should—be provided by **DAYLIGHT POWER**.

THERMOSOLAR® has Non-Imaging Optical systems which collects daylight on dull days as well as fine days to produce **FREE usable heat** (thermal energy, high temperatures) to **save 20% energy** by heating domestic hot water, space heating, industrial process heat and cooling systems.

Thermosolar® Non-Imaging Optical Systems are cost effective and suitable for District Heating, schools, hotels, apartments, public buildings, military establishments, private houses and shopping malls.

About the Author

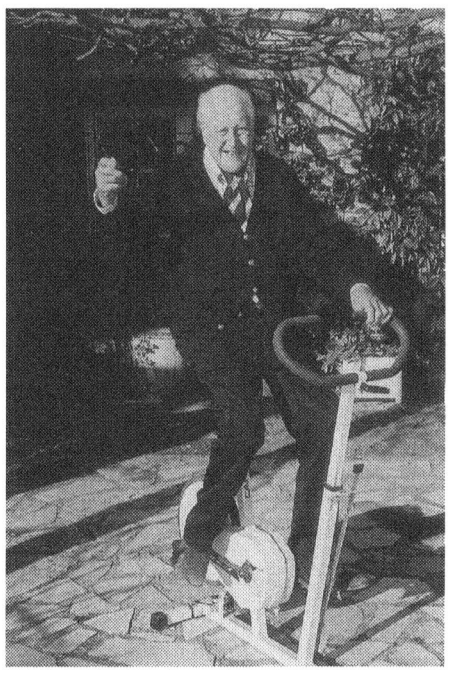

We hope that *ASCULAPIUS, Your Owner's Manual* sparks this kind of enthusiasm in our readers, and shows them how much all of us can learn about ageing, not only from books such as this one, but from the intelligence and wisdom of John H. Millar, a centenarian who has lived a long, enjoyable, passionate and healthy life.

His fascination for aviation led him to become both a British and an American pilot in the 1930s, also an Honorary Captain with American Transcontinental Airlines. In addition, he founded several dollar-earning aerospace companies in the United States and in Europe. He was a Lieutenant Commander, R.N.V.R. during WWII.

A passion for sailing enabled him to cruise in both the Atlantic and Pacific Oceans. His concern for the environment has encouraged him to create Daylight Energy Foundation, of which he is the President and has patented THERMOSOLAR, a device that collects daylight and converts it to high temperature heat.

He is a Senior Member of the Royal Yacht Squadron, a Senior Liveryman of the second Senior Company, the Worshipful Company of Grocers and a Senior Member of the Royal Aeronautical Society.

Today he is enjoying life with his wife Joanna in Monaco and on the French Riviera—his first wife, (American) the mother of his two children, died in 1962.

About the "Originator"

John Humphrey Millar, in his **hundred and three years** of life, has had a rare and impressive multi-faceted career—his knowledge acquired over more than 100 years has enabled him to share his experiences with others.

His father died when he was only 6 years old. His mother never remarried. As a result, J.H. Millar had to tackle life without a father to turn to and left school at 17 and a half, learned typing and secretarial skills and had a job in marketing, advertising and public relations.

Due to his enthusiasm, he developed the ability to overcome obstacles and attain many accomplishments in both Europe and America throughout his life.

His fascination for aviation included a British flying certificate gained in 1934. He was granted an American Pilot's Licence in New York in 1936. In 1937 he was invited to become an Honorary Captain with American Transcontinental Airlines.

In addition, he founded several dollar-earning aerospace companies employing English, Americans and Europeans, became a Lieutenant-Commander, R.N.V.R. during WWII, created and operated the only Royal Naval Air Transport Service in Southern India and Ceylon.

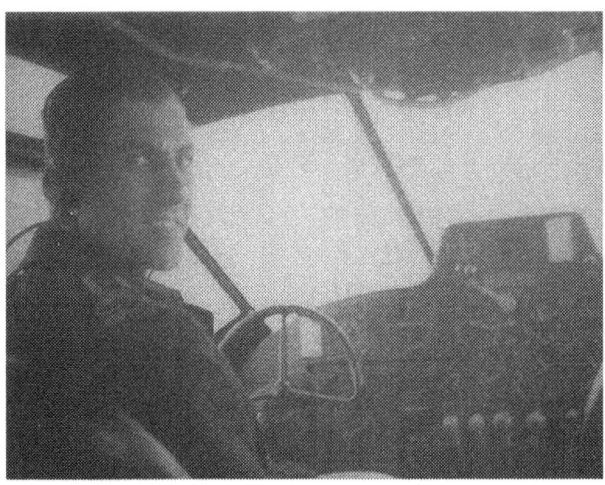

LT—CDR J.H. MILLAR RNVR at controls of "Fox Roger 880".

In January 1965, the British Prime Minister with a majority of 4 seats in the House of Commons destroyed The British Aircraft Industry. Mr Millari's English company *Avica Equipment Limited*, employing 550 people in 3 factories, lost 85 % of their order book overnight.

He therefore sold his country house in England, emigrated to Europe to work on the same clock-time. By personal contact he obtained large contracts from European customers, which saved the employment of his work people.
He was the only member of the British Aircraft Industry to organise in Europe a multi-lingual sales and engineering group which obtained substantial contracts for *Avica's* products from the European Aerospace and Nuclear Research Industries. His English and Continental European businesses were bought in 1980, when he was 77 years old, by an English public company.

The widespread pollution from burning fossil fuels encouraged him to design and develop his thermo solar device using Non-Imaging Optics to collect daylight and convert it to high temperature heat. He founded a non-profit organization—Daylight Energy Foundation—to save the ecology of the world. Also he has been a member for at least 40 years of the World Wild Trust founded by H.R.H Prince Bernhard of the Netherlands, and today WWF.

Today he is enjoying life with his wife Joanna in Monaco and on the French Riviera—his first wife, (American) the mother of his two children, died in 1962.

A passion for sailing and sail boats (33 meter Brigantine) enabled him to cruise in both the Atlantic and Pacific Oceans. He is a senior member of the Royal Yacht Squadron.

As soon as he can overcome an eye problem he will sail again in the **Oceans of the World.**

Photographs of J.H. Millar

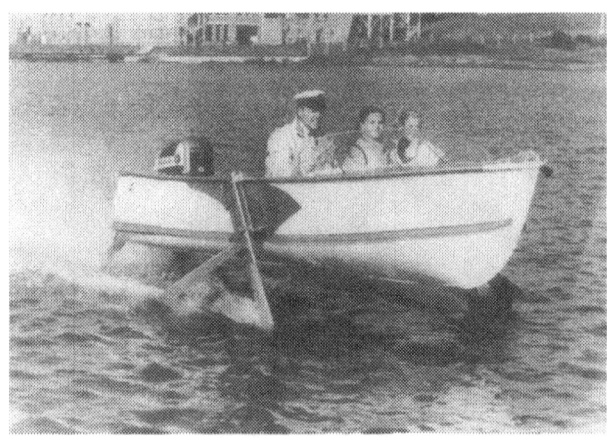

1957—The first HYDROFOIL with retractable foils at 35 knots in the Medina River, Isle of Wight.

John Humphrey Millar brought the first Hydrofoil to England. It had retractable surface piercing foils. He demonstrated in the Thames in front of the House of Commons to the Government. The Army and Royal Marines both wanted a larger size which was available but the Government refused to order them.

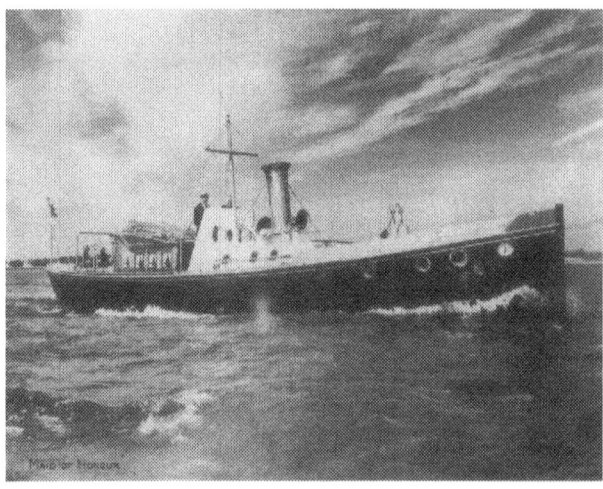

1958—The last Admiral's Barge with Brass Funnel as a tender to the challenger for the America's Cup.

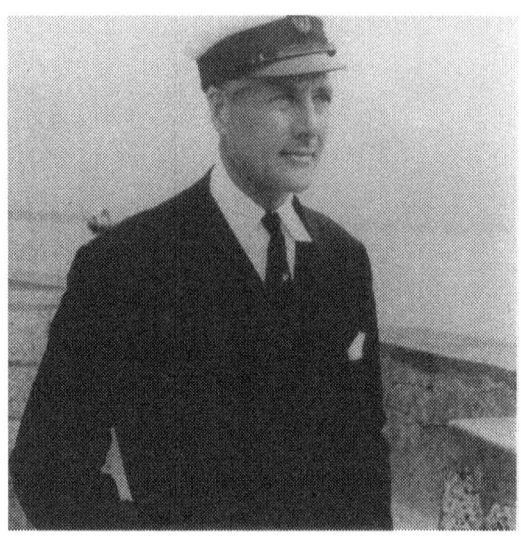

John Humphrey MILLAR

978-0-595-39138-7
0-595-39138-9